Published by Breastfeeding & Beyond Publishing
~Where evidence and tenderness belong together~

For permission requests, please contact:
Breastfeeding & Beyond
Bella Vista NSW, Australia
www.breastfeedingandbeyond.com.au

ISBN: 978-1-7643183-1-0

Cover design: Melody Jackson

Printed in Australia / Distributed worldwide via Amazon KDP

Acknowledgment of Country

This book was written on Dharug Country, where stories have been held and handed on long before mine. With gratitude to the Bidjigal people and to all Dharug Elders — past and present — and with respect to all Aboriginal and Torres Strait Islander peoples. I acknowledge that sovereignty was never ceded.

I pay particular respect to the women and mothers who have carried language, care, and culture across generations — who birth, feed, and raise children on Country.

Always was, always will be.

Author's Note

This book was written in the quiet margins of motherhood — in clinic rooms, on night feeds, between moments of work and wonder.

These poems and reflections grew from what I witness every day as a mother and a doctor: the way tenderness and evidence can belong together, how love and loss often share the same space, and how the smallest gestures of care can hold immense power.

Tender Thresholds is for anyone standing at the doorway between who they were and who they're becoming. I hope it meets you gently — wherever you are in your story.

Content Note

This book includes references to pregnancy loss, birth trauma, domestic violence, infant illness and loss, parental illness, medical procedures, and the emotional impacts of care.

Please take gentle care as you read. Pause or skip sections as needed. If difficult feelings arise, consider reaching out to a trusted person or local supports in your community.

Your wellbeing matters.

Dedication

For every mother at the threshold — those with arms full, arms empty, and those who mother in other ways.

For the little ones who were held for a moment and forever.

And for Zayn and Meryem, my greatest teachers.

Table of Contents

Prologue		9
Part I:	Becoming	10
Part II:	The Everyday Sacred	22
Part III:	Liquid Gold	36
Part IV:	Care and Consent	50
Part V:	Milk and Medicine	66
Part VI:	Shadows and Strength	86
Part VII:	Loss and Longing	108
Part VIII:	Bearing Witness	122
Part IX:	Love, With Sleeves Rolled Up	136
Part X:	The People Beside Her	146
Part XI:	Love That Outlasts	162
Part XII:	Other Ways Home	178
Part XII:	The Long Letting Go	194
Part XIV:	Milk, Power and Motherhood	208
Epilogue		231
Acknowledgements		232
About the Author		233
Further Support and Resources		234

Prologue

Motherhood is not a single threshold.
It is a thousand doorways,
a rhythm of sustenance and surrender,
of holding on and letting go.
It is joy and ache braided together,
grief and laughter coexisting in the same breath.

This is not just my story as a mother.
It is also the story I have witnessed again and again -
in clinic rooms, in waiting rooms, in whispered confessions,
in the way mothers arrive with arms full, or not,
or with hearts heavy with love that has nowhere to go.

These are fragments, meditations, truths.
Not one mother's voice, but many.
A book of thresholds,
of tenderness,
of love.

Every story of motherhood begins with a doorway:
One we step through without knowing who we will become.

Part I

Becoming

Birth makes more than a baby.
It remakes the mother too.

0 → 1

The world split open the moment you arrived.
Time bent; days blurred; I was remade.
I learned the rhythm of your breaths
before I knew myself again.
You were my first everything—
my undoing,
my anchor,
my wild new beginning.
You made me a mother.
Not because I suddenly knew how,
but because you arrived,
and I learned
in the fumbling,
the watching,
the aching,
that love does not ask
for perfection,
only presence.

1 → 2

I thought my heart was already full.
Then you came, and you did not just enter a home.
You entered a story already in motion.
And my heart stretched in ways I didn't know it could.
I missed the quiet of two,
even as I welcomed the chorus of three.
I hold one hand, then the other—
and still, somehow, I am holding them both.
I feared there would not be enough of me left to give.
I feared I would lose myself in the noise.
But instead, I found a new self—
a mother with two hands full,
a heart stretched wider,
a love without borders.
And you taught me—
love is not a pie, but a river.
It does not slice itself thinner;
it multiplies.

$2 \to \infty$

Motherhood multiplies but never divides.
We added another chair
and the table felt right.
Each child rewrites the story,
remakes the mother;
each birth
a new version of myself.
Each child carves new places in my heart,
softens the edges
I thought were fixed,
teaches me how to stretch myself beyond
the borders I once called my limits.
Home stretched without tearing—
a house with lights on in more windows.
Motherhood is paradox.
I am scattered and gathered,
tired and whole,
small and infinite,
all at once.
Motherhood does not make you once.
It makes you, and unmakes you,
and makes you again, forever.

Before You

Before you, I was whole
in ways I did not question.
After you, I discovered pieces of myself
I had never met before.
It is strange to feel both
more fragile
and more complete,
to ache with exhaustion
yet glow with a light
I never carried alone.

Explosions

You came into my life
like dawn breaking open—
not quietly,
but with an explosion of colour
and starlight,
scattering joy into corners
I didn't know were dark.
Your laughter paints the air,
your steps leave bright threads
for me to follow.
When you dance,
the whole world bends closer,
as if to learn
how light can take form
in a child.
And when you curl against me,
still small enough to fit,
I know—
I carry a universe
in the shape of you.

Teachers

I thought I was here to guide you,
but it is you who teaches me:
to slow,
to soften,
to stay present.
You slow me to watch dust dance
in the sun strip on the rug.
You name the magpie;
I learn to hear morning.
Crumbs become constellations
we sweep together.
When toast burns,
you say, "Try again,"
and we do.
You make me braver
by asking for stories,
so I soften my voice
and stay.
You make me
more human,
more fragile,
more whole.

On Becoming

Motherhood is not a single arrival,
but a thousand thresholds.
The first cry,
the first step,
the first letting go.
Each one costs me something—
and gives me something back
I never knew I was missing.
Motherhood is holding close,
and then loosening,
again and again.
A dance of tethering and release,
until the day they can stand
without my arms
and still feel the shape
of my embrace.

Full Circle

I began thinking motherhood
was something I would master.
Now I know—
it is not a task,
but a becoming.
Each day remakes me,
each child remakes me,
each story brings me back to myself.

Nanna

I was there, already forming—
an egg inside your daughter,
inside you—
a small future held
in your warmth.

You weren't famous.
But you were everything.
The bee's knees.
The hum of love
that never needed applause.

Your kitchen
was the way things
were meant to be.
Sunlight on red laminate.
Tea and pumpkin scones.
The deep freeze stacked
with papers and promise.

You never needed to be loud
to be heard.
Kindness was your language,
spoken in home cooked meals,
folded washing,
the soft press of a hand.

You taught me
that love is stronger than death.
That grief changes shape
but never disappears.

Now, when I hold a newborn,
or a mother's hand
in the midst of chaos,
I know I'm channeling
your patience,
your quiet acceptance.

You taught me that deep peace
and deep presence
can smell like roast chicken,
can sound like talkback radio,
can live in the way you listen.

Your life didn't change the world,
but it changed me.
And that is enough.

When I hold my children,
I catch glimpses of you —
the gentleness that steadied me,
the patience I'm still learning.
You are the quiet in my voice,
the light that softens
what could have hardened.

The thread
that began with you
runs on—
through my hands,
into theirs,
a quiet lineage
of love in motion.

Part II

The Everyday Sacred

The sacred hides in repetition.
The act of doing small things,
and doing them well.

Small Moon

The lamp made a small moon over the cot.
The kettle clicked;
the house learned our hush.
I counted your breaths the way
I once counted hours.
Milk warmed my shoulder;
your fingers found my thumb.
We lived between nappies
and new names for love.
I didn't know how—
only that you were here.
I swayed the hallway
thin with patience,
showing up,
until showing up
became knowing.

Night Watch

There is a holiness in hours
no one else sees.
The chair creaks;
the floor remembers.
I whisper your name
to keep the dark gentle,
and prayers
that only you
will ever hear.
Outside,
a river of sleeping windows;
we float—
where love hums
louder than silence.

The Weight of Laundry

The basket mocks me—
overflowing, relentless.
In the corner:
a tower of blocks, a squeal of delight.
I once drowned in the undone,
naming failures.
Now I read the mess
as footnotes of a day
well-lived:
Nutella on cuffs,
grass on knees,
steam on glass.
I fold what I can
and bless what I can't.

Becoming Soft

You have softened me,
sanded the edges
I thought were fixed.
I used to strive to be sharp.
Now I am glad to be rounded—
gentled,
made new.
I would rather be
gentle
than right.
Let the world rub me
smooth as riverstone—
fit for small palms,
warm with use.

What You Teach Me

I thought I was here to guide you;
you are the one teaching me—
how to linger in wonder,
how to laugh at small things,
how to forgive quickly,
how love is always an action
before it is word.

Parts of Me

Motherhood sets
a long table inside me.
The Protector watches the door;
the Pleaser pours tea.
The Critic counts the spoons;
the Child asks for a story.
They quarrel,
then soften—
someone whispers,
we're safe now.
I pass the bread,
steadying us all,
and name us whole:
a chorus,
never meant
to be one voice.

The Weight of a Hand

Your hand in mine is its own universe—
sticky with nutella,
warm with sleep,
certain.
Curling into trust.
I never want to forget your smallness,
how your fingers wrap around mine,
anchoring me to this moment.
One day your hand will pull away,
reaching for independence,
for doors I cannot enter.
But for now—
your hand is my reminder
to slow down,
to notice the gift of now.
To carry this weight
as the treasure it is.
It makes me light.

Altars in the Ordinary

Altars appear everywhere once you are here—
a highchair tray,
a laundry line,
the coffee table cluttered with toys.
We lay down offerings:
crusts,
crayons,
sighed-out air.
Sometimes I feel suffocated by it,
drowning in all that is undone.
But then—
a hand slips into mine,
a child climbs into my lap,
a sleepy head presses against my shoulder.
Suddenly the mess is not failure,
but evidence of life,
lived fully.
Evidence of love filling every corner.
The work never ends,
but perhaps that is the point.
The mess means we are alive.

Efficiency

I remind myself
I'm not a machine.
My worth isn't measured
in tasks cleared
before someone calls "Mum?"

Some days run smooth—
brief,
tidy victories.

Most days are crooked—
spills,
tears,
half-finished
thoughts,
the quiet mending
of small things.

Still,
I matter.
Not for output,
but for being here—
loving,
listening,
showing up
bone-tired
and human.

Rest, I tell myself.
I'm already enough.

The Inner Weather

Some days
I wake calm,
the whole house inside me
quiet.

Other days
everything shifts—
old storms rumble,
new worries crowd,
the air tight
before I've even risen.

I still make breakfast
for all my selves:
the tired one,
the hopeful one,
the one who wants to run,
the one who stays.

Motherhood is this—
tending the inner weather
as faithfully
as the children
at my feet.

The Clock

The clock ticks louder since you arrived.
Minutes stretch
like wet washing on the line.
I try to hold time still
and end up holding you.
We count to twenty,
then to sleep.
Let the dishes wait;
let this breath stay.
I will be late to everything
but you.

Letter to the Mother in the Middle of the Mess

I see the dishes stacked like arguments.
I see the floor learning a new language of crumbs.
You think the house is weighing your worth; it isn't—
it knows you're keeping weather over hearts.
Drink water.
Eat something from a real plate.
Ask for help before asking permission.
Hold the baby,
or yourself,
or both.
Nothing essential is late.
These ordinary, holy minutes are doing
their quiet work.
The rest can wait its turn.

Part III

Liquid Gold

Feeding is not only nourishment.
It is communication made flesh.

Memory Made Liquid

Milk is not just milk,
but memory made liquid.
The body remembering
how to give,
how to soften,
how to keep a child alive
with nothing more
than its own letting go.

The World Becomes Smaller

In the dark,
her cry folds the night in half.
You gather her close,
skin against skin,
and the world becomes smaller—
only this breath,
only this mouth,
only this milk
passing between us.

The Silken Thread

Breastfeeding is a tether—
not a chain,
but a silken thread.
Invisible,
except for the way it keeps
two hearts
from drifting
too far from one another.

The First Language

At the breast
a child learns the world is kind.
Warmth meets hunger,
comfort answers need.
It is a first language,
spoken without words:
I am here,
you are safe,
love can be swallowed whole.

Medals of Devotion

Milk stains on a shirt,
damp crescents of devotion.
No one claps for these,
yet they are medals—
quiet proofs
that a mother's body
has poured itself out
to keep another body
growing.

Startled by the Gift

I never thought
my body could do this—
make milk,
make comfort,
make a rhythm
that soothed you back into sleep.
Each latch still startles me:
you ask, I give,
and the world feels
possible again.

The Quiet Revolution

We have fed our babies
in kitchens,
on buses,
in waiting rooms where eyes
looked away.
We have fed them in secret,
and in pride.
Breastfeeding is the
quiet revolution
of ordinary women
saying with our bodies:
every child
deserves enough.

Worth the Giving

There were nights
when I wanted to stop—
my skin sore,
my chest aching.
But then you looked at me,
milk still shining on your lip,
and I remembered:
love is not always easy,
but it is always,
always
worth the giving.

Prayer and Promise

We know the weight of a
hungry cry,
the relief of milk
letting down.
We know the power of small mouths
to draw not just sustenance,
but hope.
Breastfeeding is not only food—
it is prayer,
and promise,
and survival.

More than Numbers

The world tells me to measure—
millilitres,
minutes,
percentiles,
charts.
But you remind me
that growth is not
only numbers.
It is the way your hand
rests open on my chest,
the way your eyes flutter closed,
trusting I will
never leave you empty.

The Milky Way

Milk is a galaxy—
rivers of light
spilled across a small mouth,
stars scattered in the dark
between your breath and mine.
Each let-down a constellation,
each swallow a comet
tracing its arc
through the silence of night.
You anchor me
to this universe
of skin and warmth,
of hunger met
and love unmeasured.
The Milky Way
is not far above us.
It is here,
flowing from my body
into yours.

Drinking the Sun

I, your baby, do not know words yet—
only warmth,
only scent,
only the rhythm of you.
The world is too bright,
too loud,
too new—
but here,
against your skin,
the light softens.
Milk pools at the corner of my mouth,
and I drink the sun.
It tastes like safety,
like the hum of your heart,
like home returning.
I do not know that you laboured
to make this gold.
I only know
that it comes when I call,
that it quiets the storm,
that it teaches me
what enough feels like.
And though my eyes are closed,
I see you—
the glow around your body,
the halo of us,
as day begins again.

Part IV

Care & Consent

The work of medicine is not only technical.
It is relational, embodied, sacred.

Consent

"Is this touch okay?"
I ask,
and wait.
Not the quick yes—
the yes that feels like one.
Your shoulders lower a fraction.
We name what comes next.
We move at the speed of safety.

Hands

I wash mine slowly,
on purpose—
warm water,
quiet foam.
A small ritual before your skin.
Clean, sure,
but gentle—
as if the sink is watching.

The Examination

We sit first.
We talk first.
Then I ask again—
"Still okay?"
You nod.
I narrate each step,
so your body hears the plan
before my hands do.

Language

We use the right words,
and the soft ones too.
Nipple, breast, latch—
also:
comfort,
warmth,
rest.
Anatomy meets mercy,
in the same sentence.

Names for Pain

You say "it stings,"
then "burns,"
then "like glass."
We gather words like clues.
Pain named
is pain already moving.
I write it down carefully,
so the chart does not argue with your body.

Safety

Door open.
Chair by the window.
Your partner on your chosen side.
You keep your shirt on—
we work around dignity.
Nothing hidden,
nothing rushed.
Let the room
steady.
No fixing.
No urgency.
Just presence—
quiet,
anchored,
unshaken.
Capacity grows
when pressure falls.
The baby learns safety
by watching us.

Chaperone

Another set of eyes,
kind ones.
A witness who brings light
just by standing there.
Sometimes safety
is a person in the corner
with steady hands
and time.

Evidence & Tenderness

Numbers help.
So do tissues.
We try the tool,
the technique,
stop if it hurts,
switch if it doesn't help.
Care is a study of one,
replicated daily.
Your relief is the result
that matters.

Boundaries

Yes to comfort,
no to urgency.
Yes to questions,
no to "just relax."
Your body is the expert;
we are the guests.
I ask before I connect—
and I thank you when I leave.

Not Yet

You don't have a yes today.
That's still a kind of knowing.
We pause.
We choose the path
that waits with you.
Trust grows slow—
like milk,
like morning.

Discharge

We stand.
You breathe.
I hand you paper that won't hold the whole story.
But it holds enough—
steps,
names,
a map for the dark.
Follow up: soon.
Hope: sooner.

Note to Self (Doctor)

Be the gentlest thing in the room.
Speak last.
Apologise quickly.
Chart with care;
someone will live inside these words.
Hold the line on safety.
Hold the person
more than the plan.

Be the Guide, Not the Guru

You walk into the room
the doctor,
the expert,
thinking you
need to know
everything
before you even
sit down.

But listen—
healing has never asked
for mastery.

The nervous system
doesn't soften
for expertise.
It softens
for presence.

You don't need to fix
what someone else
has carried
for a lifetime.

You don't need to
stitch together
stories that aren't
yours to hold.

Sit.
Be here.
Let the air settle.

Trust is built
in the small spaces—
the unclenched jaw,
the honest pause,
the moment you admit
you don't know
but you're willing to stay.

We are not above
the people we help.
We are beside them.
Human to human.

This is the beginning
of another kind of medicine.
Two nervous systems,
meeting without armour,
walking the terrain together—
not as expert
and wounded,
but as companions
charting a way forward
one steady breath
at a time.

Part V

Milk & Medicine

Science explains the body.
Tenderness teaches us how to heal it.

Clinic Morning

Keys in the door.
Kettle on.
The room remembers how to
hold people.
I wipe down the chair,
straighten the artwork,
and promise the walls
we'll be gentle.

The Order of Care

We start with names.
Then stories.
Then bodies.
Order matters—
language first,
so the nervous system can hear
us coming.

Milk and medicine,
both require permission.
Both ask:
May I touch?
May I know?
May I help you carry this?

We do not rush the body.
We let it arrive in its own time.
Because healing begins
not at the breast
or the prescription pad,
but in the quiet moment
someone says your name
and waits for you to answer.

Latch Notes

Mouth wide.
Chin soft.
Bodies talking in a grammar older than charts.
We adjust a shoulder,
unlearn some "shoulds,"
wait for the sigh that means yes.

This is not just mechanics—
it's memory and mammal,
instinct meeting instruction.

The nipple brushes the lip,
a question without words.
The baby answers
with a root,
a lean,
a reaching.

We pause for breath,
not correction.
Hands hover,
listening
more than leading.

Milk is waiting.
But first—
alignment,
trust,
the quiet recalibration
of two nervous systems
trying to meet in the middle.

Mastitis

Heat that bites.
Red that worries.
We cool,
we rest,
we plan.

Anti-inflammatories,
fluids,
watch for the fevers that don't back down.

The ache is sharp,
but so is the
loneliness
of not being heard.

Relief is also treatment.
So is asking,
How are you really?
So is being believed.

Pumping

Not penance.
A tool.
We choose
flange,
pace,
breaks,
hospital-grade or hand-held.

You whisper
not enough.

But it's not milk
that's scarce—
it's trust
in a body
told to doubt itself.

We measure,
we breathe,
we slow the room
together.

Your shoulders drop—
that's data too.
Milk is more than volume;
so are you.

Millilitres are not
how you measure
worth.

Relactation

Any milk is a win.
We say it out loud.
Skin to skin.
Small goals,
kind clocks.
Syringe,
spoon,
pump,
breast—
there is no wrong door back in.

You surprise yourself—
the body remembers,
and sometimes,
forgives.

Scales

Numbers are a language,
not a verdict.
We read them in context,
as one part of the picture,
against charts and curves,
but never against the mother.

We weigh the baby—
and everything else lightly.
Birth weight.
Discharge weight.
Percentiles rising, dipping,
the dotted line we follow
but never let become the whole map.

We note the grams gained,
the millilitres taken,
feeds per twenty-four hours,
nappies wet or dry—
because data has its place.
But so does the way
she holds her breath
while the digits settle.
So does the way
the baby melts into her chest
after the feed.

We chart the numbers,
but we also chart the story.
Because growth is more than a line,
and health is more than a percentile.

Postnatal Depression

Weight that lingers.
Fog that worries.

We screen,
we ask,
we pause.
Sleep,
nutrition,
watch for the
darkness
that doesn't lift.

The drag is real,
but so is the
silence
around her struggle.

Validation is treatment,
too.
So is saying,
This looks hard.

So is staying long enough
to hear
what she nearly
didn't say.

This work is gentle:
naming the fog,
holding the edges
so she doesn't fall through them.

Medications

We talk through options.
What helps,
what risks,
what fits your life.

Side effects,
supply,
half-lives—
what it does to milk,
what it does to you.

You choose.
Autonomy is a dose
we prescribe early.

All the Advice

Water.
Food.
Rest if you can
(and if you can't, we plan).
Ignore the chorus of "should."
Keep the voices that are kind.
The rest
can wait outside.

Evidence & Tenderness

Numbers in one hand,
tissues in the other.
Trial.
Notice.
Adapt.
Care is a study of one,
replicated daily.
We measure.
We feel.
We listen.
Your ease
is the outcome.

The Myth of "Fine"

"How are you?"
"I'm fine."
But I have learned to hear
the truth behind the word.
Fine is often code
for bone-deep loneliness,
for tears shed in the shower,
for "I need help":
left unsent.

Notes for the Night Shift

I write like someone will live here—
because you will.
Plain words,
no heroics.
Findable at 2 a.m.,
when the light is dim
and the house is loud with quiet.

I write so you won't have to guess
what I meant
or what mattered.

Just enough light
to carry you
through the doorway
of the next decision.

Home Visit

Shoes by the door.
Toast in the air.
We weigh
on the kitchen bench,
between crayons
and courage.
Notes beside the kettle,
breast pump
on the couch.
Your dog watches every move
like it matters—
because it does.

The plan fits better
when it smells like your house,
when the baby is held
in their own light.
Care lands softer here—
where medicine sits
next to the fruit bowl.

When It's Hard

We pause.
Door open.
Partner close.
Breath first.
Nothing rushed.
Tears allowed.
Lights low if needed.
We choose the next smallest step
that feels like yes.

Not perfect—
just possible.
And that is enough.

You Are Enough

At first,
it feels impossible—
to unclench,
to soften,
to trust that the world
will not collapse
if you stop holding it up.

But then—
a breath,
a sigh,
a warmth unfurling from the centre.
The jaw loosens,
shoulders sink,
the chest becomes a tide.

This is what the body remembers
when the mind finally quiets:
that milk flows
only when we stop trying,
that rest is not weakness
but wisdom.

To relax
is to return—
to the small steady rhythm
of being enough,
right now,
just as you are.

The Slow Medicine Collective

In every corner
of this work
I find them—
doctors who choose
the slow road,
the soft road,
the human road.

No headlines.
No glamour.
Just rooms
where mothers
finally breathe.

They hold stories
with steady hands:
pain,
trauma,
milk tangled
in fear
or memory
or hope.

They know
feeding is never "just feeding",
that every dyad
carries whole worlds,
that healing
never hurries.

They stay curious.
Stay tender.
Stay human
in systems built
for speed.

This community—
scattered,
yet united
by belief in
mother and child,
in physiology,
in compassion—
is the quiet backbone
of breastfeeding medicine.

They remind us
what care becomes
when science
and softness
learn to walk
together.

Part VI

Shadows & Strength

Even when safety falters and joy thins,
mothers carry light no one
taught them to hold.

The Past We Carry

Some mothers begin
already haunted.
Not by spirits,
but by touch withheld,
by rooms that were not safe.

The past does not vanish
just because a baby
is placed in our arms.
It lingers—
in shoulders that flinch,
in breath held too long.

Love does not cancel history.
It lives beside it.
And still—
I have seen mothers
hold their child
as if no one ever held them.

And here is a softer truth:
love can travel backwards.
In holding a child,
some part of us is held, too.
Not erased—
but rewritten,
with gentler hands.

Generational Echoes

Some wounds are inherited,
passed quietly down the line.
Still, I've seen mothers
stand like trees in the storm,
hands trembling,
voice soft but present,
choosing to plant something different.

The past doesn't disappear.
It shifts.
Roots deepen.
Branches shelter.
And what was once only survival
begins to sound a little more
like love.

After the Comment

It was said lightly—
routine,
nothing meant by it.

But your body heard
something else.
Old alarm
waking fast.

The room stayed the same.
Your pulse didn't.
You nodded,
answered politely,
did everything right—
on the outside.

Inside,
the past was suddenly
too close.

No one saw
the way your breath shrank
to a corner of your ribs.

Later,
you couldn't explain
why you were shaking.

There were no new wounds—
just an old one,
brushed against
by accident.

Dissociation

"Just relax,"
they said.
Meaning well.
Not knowing.

But those words
have lived before—
in rooms
with no softness,
no choice.

Your jaw tightened.
You left your body
to stay in the room.
Because that is how
you learned
to survive.

They moved on,
charting vitals.
They had no idea
how loud it can get
in the quiet.

You breathed in pieces,
quietly stitching yourself
back into your skin.

First Mother

She was adopted—
raised with love,
but no map
for where she came from.

She says it like a footnote—
nothing urgent,
just background.

Now she holds her baby,
her mirror,
and doesn't know
how close to stand.

They tell her
hold the child
skin to skin,
let love arrive.

But skin
was never a safe language.
She wants to want this
more easily.

Her arms know how to hold,
but her heart
hesitates at the door.

Everyone says
it will come.
Maybe it will—
because love, for her,
is something learned,
not inherited.

And so,
each day she tries:
the baby's head
against her chest,
her silence slowly
making room
for a yes.

Still trying.
That is a kind of
medicine, too.

A lineage of touch
being relearned.

A mother healing the story
of her own birth.

Startle Reflex

The baby cries
and my body
is already running—
before my mind
catches up.

No danger, I say.
Just need, and sound.
But my pulse
doesn't listen.
I hate that the past can reach me here.

Some nights
I hold her close
and still feel far away,
as if love must travel
through fog to find me.

She doesn't know
the ghosts behind my calm—
only the steadiness
of arms that keep returning.

And maybe
that is enough—
that I stay,
even when
my body
wants to flee.
The quiet, persistent
choosing
to begin again.

Birth Trauma

Birth is supposed to be a threshold
into joy,
but sometimes it is a wound.
Bodies cut,
voices unheard,
fear flooding where safety
should have been.

Some mothers
speak of their births
as battles they
barely survived.
And then they are expected
to smile,
to pose for photos,
to nurse at breasts
still trembling
with shock.

Trauma lingers
in the scar that aches years later,
in the heart that races
at the sound of alarms.

But I have also seen healing—
when she is believed
when pain is named,
when strength is honoured
instead of denied.

Flat Line

Everything
is functioning.

Feeds happen.
Clothes are clean.
Smiles
appear
when required.

But inside,
it's all
grey noise.
No rise,
no fall—
just the hum
of getting through.

They said
it would lift.
I keep waiting
for light
to mean something again.

The baby laughs.
I know
it's beautiful.
I just
can't feel it
yet.

Still,
each morning,
I get up.
Each feed,
I reach out.

Maybe love
isn't a flood.

Maybe
it's a slow drip—
drop
by drop,
life returning.

Motherhood, Underwater

The baby is here.
Everyone says
"you must be so happy."

She nods,
because the truth
feels too heavy
to hold in front of them.

Days blur—
baby vomit on her shirt,
feeds that melt
into each other,
a tiredness that isn't
just tiredness
but something darker
pooling under her ribs.

She loves her baby.
That part is steady.
But love and despair
can sit in the same room,
breathing the same air.

She waits
for the "rush"
everyone promised,
as if joy arrives
on a timetable.

Instead—
she feels like she's underwater,
moving through thick,
soundless days,
watching the world
from behind glass.

Small tasks
become mountains:
a shower,
a sandwich,
the first step
out the door.

But she tells someone—
or someone notices.
And slowly,
a hand reaches in.

The fog doesn't lift at once.
It thins.
It softens.
Moments of light
break through
like small, stubborn seeds.

Rebuilding isn't a leap.
It's a series
of barely noticeable steps
into colour.

And in time
she finds her way
back to herself—
still a mother,
still tender,
but no longer lost
in the dark.

Tick Boxes

The checklist says
"mood stable."
The chart says
"bonding adequate."
But healing
rarely fits
the tick-box lines.

I watch
how she lifts the baby—
gentle, efficient,
a nurse's precision
without the joy.
This is not absence.
It's survival.

So instead of
how are you feeling,
I ask,
how are you managing to keep going?

Her eyes well.
She exhales.
For the first time,
she lets herself be seen.

I write
"follow-up in two weeks."
What I mean is:
hope is still here,
quietly breathing
beneath the surface.

Courage, Chosen

Trauma teaches us to leave ourselves,
to escape when life feels unbearable.
Doors that were nailed shut years ago
can get flung right open.

And yet – I see mothers stay.
Here, in their skin.
In their bodies,
in the moment,
with their babies.
Sometimes their hands
not quite steady,
sometimes tears fall
unchecked.

But still,
these mothers choose
to rock,
to feed,
to comfort.
This is not small.
It is not easy,
this defiance against
the past.

It is survival
turned into love.
It is the quiet courage
that remakes the world.
It is love,
rewriting the story
through skin.

Clinic Notes (Unwritten)

She smiles
when I ask
how the birth was.
Says,
"It was fine."
Then pauses—
too long.

I see her eyes
flicker to the floor,
her hands tighten
on the pram handle.

Her notes say
postpartum recovery:
uneventful.
Trauma
rarely makes it into
discharge summaries.

She talks about
feeding,
fatigue,
stitches that still pull.

I listen
for what isn't said—
for the tremor
beneath ordinary words.

When she tells me
she slept
without dreaming,
I write,
"Improved rest."
What I mean is:
her body
is starting
to believe
she's safe.

I see.
She is not fragile.
She is fierce.
Post-traumatic stress,
the diagnosis reads.
But what I witness
is *post-traumatic love*—
the daily, deliberate
act of staying.

There is no billing code
for that.

Just quiet awe
that fills the room
each time she holds her baby
and does not turn away.

Returning

The climb back
isn't dramatic—
no sudden light,
just a slow loosening
of the tight places.

Some mornings now,
she sleeps
without scanning the dark.

Other times she still breaks—
suddenly,
sharply.

But now
she knows how
to gather herself,
how to breathe
until the pieces
hold again.

And the child—
growing,
laughing,
reaching for her
with absolute trust—
becomes a reminder
that she is more
than what was
done to her.

One quiet afternoon
she catches her reflection
with the baby on her hip
and sees someone steadier,
someone softened,
someone returning
to herself.

Healing looks like
sun instead of shadow,
touch that lands softly,
Being held without
bracing for impact.

She is not finished healing.
She may never be
fully unmarked.

But she is living now
on her own terms—
and that,
after everything,
is its own kind
of homecoming.

Becoming

Healing doesn't happen
in straight lines.
it's a spiral
back through memory,
each visit
a small reclamation.

It happens
in tiny permissions:
I can hold him.
I can soothe her.
I can stay present.
I am safe now.

Over time,
her body learns
a new language—
one she writes
with her child:
truth without threat,
love without fear,
touch that belongs
to her.

In this quiet
daily labour,
she becomes the parent
she never had,
and the person
she was always meant
to be.

Letter to the Mother Who Still Trembles

I see you.
You,
whose body holds memories
you never asked for.
You,
whose skin still remembers,
whose breath still quickens at the echo of old hurts.
You thought becoming a mother
might wipe the slate clean.
But here you are—
holding your baby
with trembling hands,
wondering if your history
disqualifies you
from tenderness.
Let me tell you what I have seen:
your very presence is resistance.
Every kiss you place on your baby's head
is a rebellion.
Every gentle touch
is a rewriting of history.
You are not broken.
You are a warrior carrying love
through the aftershocks.
And in the eyes of your child,
you are already enough.

Part VII

Loss & Longing

Loss is part of the landscape of care.
We honour what cannot stay by tending what remains.
Even there, especially there,
love has work to do.

The First Breath

I have watched babies take their first breath,
and mothers take their first step
into a story that will undo them
and make them whole.

Diagnoses

Some babies arrive with stories
that bend the air around them.
Syndromes,
scars,
unexpected paths.
Their mothers weep,
then rise,
then learn to carry both joy
and grief
in the same hand.
By morning they are fluent
in a new language.

They love in every tense at once.

The Baby We Never Met

Some mothers carry children
whose feet never touched the earth.
Their names live in the quiet between days—
their absence stitched into every season.
Birthdays
and weather
and song.
Grief is not measured by days,
but by the size of the love
that had no place to land
and still,
somehow,
it lands in us.

Early Loss

Two pink lines,
then silence.
The world says, move on—
as if hope can be tucked away
like a folded test in a drawer.
As if these beginnings are trivial.
But a brief beginning
is still a beginning.
And I know:
you carry what almost was—
light you saw for a moment
and will not forget.

Empty Arms

I have seen mothers
walk out of hospital with empty arms.
There is silence where a heartbeat should be.
A silence that seeps into every corner of a life.
Their bodies still aching with milk,
their hearts unbearably full of love
that has nowhere to go.
There are no right words
for this kind of leaving—
only presence,
only witness.
So we sit,
breathe,
say the name.

Perhaps love is how we carry
what we cannot keep.

After Loss

Grief does not leave—
it weaves itself into the fabric of love.
The baby is gone,
but the mother remains.

She is changed,
and that too is love.

The Baby Who Smiled for a Season

I once cared for a child
who smiled only for a season.
Her laugh filled the room like sunlight,
her parents glowing with every milestone—
first giggle,
first tooth,
a dozen ordinary joys
made luminous by fragility.
And then—
silence.
An absence so loud
it still echoes.
A family remade by love and by grief,
walking forward with
arms empty,
yet hearts forever marked
by the brief, brilliant life
of their child.
Sometimes I weep in the car
afterward,
carrying echoes of grief
that was never mine
and yet still lives in me.
Even now,
I find myself whispering her name.
We say the name softly
as if to keep it warm.
To forget would feel like betrayal.
To remember is a small act
of keeping her near.

Unimaginable

There are moments in medicine
that undo me.
When a mother looks at me,
eyes hollowed by grief,
and asks, "How do I go on?"

There is no answer.
No textbook prepares you
No protocol guides you
for the weight of a
parent's despair.
In those moments,
I am not doctor
but human.
I sit with them,
I cry with them,
I let my silence say what
words cannot.

The helplessness is unbearable.
And yet,
to witness,
to not turn away,
to stay in the room—
perhaps that is the
one small mercy
we can give.

Held in the Light

You pictured
easy—
soft cheeks,
steady milestones,
a future unfolding simply.

Instead—
genetic reports,
monitors blinking,
hands learning how to hold
without fear of breaking.
Love stays.

But it shifts shape—
into watching,
waiting,
celebrating every almost.

Grief is here too—
not for the child you hold,
but for the story
you thought you'd live.

And still,
in morning light,
their fingers find yours.
Not what you imagined.
Still holy.

The Child Not Yet Lost

There are other griefs,
the ones that come with diagnoses—
syndromes, prognoses, futures
that parents never imagined.

I have seen mothers and fathers
crumple in hospital chairs,
their faces collapsing under news
that rewrote their lives.
And I have seen them stand again,
tears still on their cheeks,
arms still outstretched
to hold their child.

Grief and love
woven together in the same breath.
Despair and devotion
coexisting in the same body.
This too is motherhood,
this too is fatherhood—
an unbreakable vow:
I will not turn away.

Rituals of Goodbye

Handprints.
Footprints.
Ink that will not wash away.
A curl of hair,
ribboned.
A hat the size of a peach.
We bathe and dress—
slow as prayer.
Photos in soft light,
softer hands.
A blanket folded into a box
none of us wanted,
now heavy with
almost.
We tuck a note,
a blessing,
say the name again.
Sometimes we plant something
that will keep reaching for light.
We teach our hands
that letting go
is also a way of holding.
The leaving has edges now;
love keeps touching them.

Letter to the Parent Whose Arms Ache

I see the ache that wakes with you and lies down at night.
You think love failed because the outcome did not change.

It did not.

Your love held as far as love could go,
and now it holds in memory,
which is also real.
Say their name when you need to.
Eat,
drink water,
step into the sun.
Put your bare feet onto the grass.
Let others carry what you cannot today.
Nothing essential is late.

Love keeps time for you.

Part VIII

Bearing Witness

Listening with the whole self.
It changes both the teller and the listener.

The Waiting Room

I have watched mothers in waiting rooms,
eyes on the floor,
hands restless in their laps.
Behind the fear is a love
so fierce,
so raw,
so relentless,
it could split the earth.
I see it—
even when they cannot.

The Doubt of Mothers

Almost every mother I meet
believes she is not enough.
Baby cries too much,
feeds too little,
sleeps too short—
and she blames herself.
I have learned to listen
between the lines.
Her doubt is proof of her care.
Her worry is proof of her love.
The very fear of failing
is evidence she isn't.
If only she could see herself as I do—
weary,
brave,
astonishingly enough.

Mirrors

In my clinic chair
I meet women who doubt,
who weep from exhaustion,
who love through fear.
They remind me daily:
motherhood is not performance—
it is presence.
I wish I could hold a mirror
and show them who they are.

Fragile Triumphs

Some babies arrive like miracles—
hearts stitched by surgeons,
lungs coaxed by machines,
tiny bodies fighting the odds.

Mothers learn courage
one fragile breath at a time.
Hands on the incubator glass,
they sing to a child
tangled in wires.
The most ordinary love,
and the most extraordinary.

I carry those faces with me—
proof that heroism
can be
quiet,
steady,
unrelenting.

Shared Stories

In clinic rooms
and waiting rooms
I hear fragments of lives.
No story the same,
each threaded with love,
fear,
courage,
surrender.
These stories
remake me.

The Thread

We are bound,
all of us—
by sleepless nights,
by whispered prayers,
by griefs
and fears
we do not name
aloud.
Motherhood is
the thread
that stitches
strangers
into kin.

Hands Open

I used to think my role
was only to help—
answers,
plans,
care.

Now I know
I am also the one who receives.
Resilience remakes me.
Tenderness remakes me.
Love remakes me.

I am not only a doctor.
I am a witness.
And that, too,
is holy work.

In Each Other

Every mother I meet
holds up a mirror.
Her story is not mine,
but I find pieces of myself in hers.
We are never truly alone
on this road.

Night Shift of the Heart

Some nights,
I hold a baby to my chest
and feel the familiar weight—
not a patient,
not a chart,
just my child
breathing trust into my collarbone.

But the part of me
that listens for trouble
never fully sleeps.
Diagnosis is a shadow
that follows me home.

In the clinic,
I cradle other people's stories—
their milk,
their fear,
their hope to be seen,
in wholeness.

I know that hope.
I carry it too.

Both

I am the hands that heal
and the hands that tremble,
the one who reassures
and the one who needs reassurance.

Mother.
Doctor.
Both.

Two hearts
beating in one body,
learning how to care
without disappearing,
learning how to stay
soft
and still strong.

Between Rooms

I change coats
and roles,
often in the same breath.
One moment,
I am the answer.
The next,
I am the one who needs holding.
Love follows me
everywhere—
I only switch
which heart
I'm tending.

Letter to the Mother in My Clinic Chair

You sit across from me,
eyes heavy.
"I think I'm not enough," you say,
and list the ways you believe you're failing—
a baby who won't sleep,
milk that feels too little,
a heart weighted with worry.
Here is what I want you to hear:
You are not failing.
You are showing up,
again and again,
inside exhaustion and doubt.
That is love.
That is motherhood.
When I look at you I see
courage stitched into nights,
tenderness poured into feeds,
resilience in every tear you swallow.
Let me hold the truth
until you can hold it for yourself:
you are already enough.
You always have been.

Part IX

Love, With Sleeves Rolled Up

Advocacy begins where endurance meets care.
It is love, practised in public.

Speaking Up

In clinic rooms I have learned
that advocacy is not loud,
but steady.
It is telling the truth,
insisting on dignity,
refusing to let a mother's pain
be brushed aside as "nothing."

The Steady Work

It is not always a speech.
Often it is persistence—
forms refilled,
calls repeated,
letters sent into quiet inboxes.
Sitting beside a mother who says,
"They told me it's in my head,"
and answering,
"No. I believe you.
We keep going."
Not glamorous.
But love,
with sleeves rolled up.

Against the Current

To advocate is to swim upstream—
against bureaucracy,
against indifference,
against a system never built
to hear mothers.
I have seen women learn new languages—
policies, protocols—
just to keep a baby safe.
Rage that shakes.
Exhaustion that buckles.
Standing again, anyway.
Love carved into petitions,
phone calls,
small brave insistences:
My child matters.
I will not be silenced.

For Our Children

There is no fiercer love
than the love that speaks for a child.
It does not flinch at institutions.
It does not shrink when told to wait.
It rises—
again and again—
even when the mother is running
on empty.
Courtrooms.
Sterile offices.
Doors that try to stay shut.
Hoarse voice,
breaking heart,
unrelenting love.
Advocacy is a mother's vow
made visible.

When Systems Fail

Referrals lost.
Symptoms dismissed.
Concerns minimised
until it is late — too late.
The face a mother makes
when she learns the net has holes—
I do not forget.
And yet—
I have watched her rise,
knock, then push, then enter,
carry her child through barriers
that should never have been there.
Her love fills the gaps
left by carelessness.
Her resilience teaches the system
to pay attention.

Hard Truths

I have stood beside mothers
who felt small before the machine—
doctors, diagnoses, desks.
Together we found words
that turned silence into motion.
It is persistent work,
this insisting on being heard.
Not because we shout,
but because we stay.

In Her Voice

Sometimes my job
is not to speak for her,
but to hand her the microphone.
To remind her:
you are the expert
on your baby,
your body,
your truth.
I have watched voices grow in real time—
from careful whisper
to steady declaration.
The moment she realises
she was never small at all—
I hold my breath,
and let the room widen.

Letter to the Mother Who Fights

I know you are tired.
Paperwork tired.
Phone-on-hold tired.
Being-polite-when-you-shouldn't-have-to tired.
You have told your story so many times
it aches to say it again.
Please hear this:
You are not difficult.
You are determined.
You are not overreacting.
You are protecting.
Drink water.
Eat something warm.
Ask one more person to stand beside you.
Let me write the letter.
Let me hold the file while you hold your child.
When they say wait—
we will mark the date,
and we will not let it drift.
Thank you for proving,
again and again,
that love, when tested,
does not break.
It learns new ways
to be strong.

Part X

The People Beside Her

The village is not a metaphor.
It is a necessity.

When Partners Falter

Postpartum is heavy work.
The body healing,
the baby feeding,
the house never still.
It is a season meant to be shared.
And yet—
too often—
she is left carrying the whole weight.
Partners step back instead of forward,
lost in their own worlds,
while she bleeds,
while she cries,
while she stitches herself together
in the dark.
This is not weakness when she weeps.
It is injustice.

The Invisible Work

The hardest work is often
the least seen.
These mothers...
they cook,
they clean,
they soothe,
they wake—
and still feel invisible.
A partner distracted,
a family absent,
a culture that calls this
"not working".
Endless lists,
a thousand tiny tasks,
the scaffolding that keeps
a family standing.
She remembers
vaccines,
nappy sizes,
which side fed last,
when the fever peaked,
what will soothe,
who needs water,
where the school form is hiding.
No clocking off.
No fanfare.
And yet—
this is the work
that holds a child's
world together.

The Loneliness of Two

There is a loneliness
that can bloom beside a person
meant to see you.
I meet mothers
cradling a baby with one arm
and their aching heart with the other.
A partner sleeps through,
scrolls through,
walks past the laundry
as if it were air.
She wonders if she asks
too much—
when all she asks
is to not be invisible.

Noticing

Some partners fade
into the background,
waiting for "when it's easier,"
for the baby to be bigger,
for the fog to lift.

But these early days matter.
The baby notices.
The mother notices.
Absence leaves a mark
as deep as presence.

When Love Steps Up

And yet—
I've seen partners step in
with both feet.
Rise at night.
Cook, clean, soothe.
"This is our baby,
this is our work,
this is our joy."
When partners show up fully,
the house exhales.
The weight halves.
Joy finds space again.
This is not "help."
It is companionship.
Love made visible.
May every mother find this—
not a helper,
but a companion
in the making of a family.

Not Alone

You were never meant
to carry all of this
by yourself.

Not the nights
that stretch too long,
not the worry
that steals your breath,
not the questions
that keep you awake
long after the baby sleeps.

There is strength
in reaching out a hand,
in saying
"Can you help?"
and letting the answer be
"Of course."

Mothering is heavy
because love is heavy.
But when we share the weight—
suddenly
it feels like something
we can hold.

Fault Lines

She walks carefully
around his moods—
not tiptoeing,
just calculating,
like stepping over cracks
only she can see.

Domestic violence isn't always
a slammed door;
sometimes it's
the soft voice
that tightens
around her choices.

He calls it love.
She calls it
keeping the peace.

Motherhood
makes the stakes sharper.
A small hand
curled in hers
anchors her to the floor
and to the future
at the same time.

She becomes an expert
in reading danger—
the hitch in his breath,
the too-long pause,
the evening quiet
that tastes metallic.

But she also becomes
an expert in hope:
stashing documents,
memorising numbers,
teaching the child
which neighbour to run to,
lifting joy
where she can find it.

Every plan she makes
is a crack of light.
Every day she stays safe
is a step
toward a different story.

People say
she should leave.
They don't see
how leaving
is crawling up a
mountain
with children on her back.

Still—
she feels the ground
shifting.
She feels herself
returning.

When she finally goes,
it will not be sudden.
It will be the slow,
steady courage
she has been gathering
for years.

Untitled (For Now)

The older child watches
too closely now,
pulls the younger one
behind her legs
when voices sharpen.

Some days
she wonders
if leaving is love.
Some days
she knows
staying is survival.

Then the children notice
how she folds herself
smaller
as she hears the key turn
in the door.

That's when she decides.

Not for herself,
though she deserves it—
but for the small bodies
learning fear
by studying hers.

And there is a spark
she guards fiercely—
a quiet promise
she makes only
to herself.

It is dark work.
Lonely work.
But she does it anyway.

One day,
she will move
in her own skin again.

One day,
the house will exhale
with her.

One day,
her children
will know
only the best version
of her.

They
will grow up
knowing
that strength
is not loudness—
it is choosing
freedom
while carrying
those you love
toward the light.

Shared Load

Motherhood was never meant to be solitary.
The village has shrunk;
partnership can be the bridge.
To share the load
is not charity.
It is justice.

Raising a child is the work of two hearts,
two sets of hands,
two lives intertwined.
When the load is shared,
a mother can rest.

She can breathe.
She can remember she is not
only mother,
but woman,
human,
whole.

He Turns the Lights On

When the night feels heavy
and her hope runs thin,
he rises first—
padding softly through the dark.
He brings water,
brings warmth,
brings steadiness.
Not trying to fix,
just staying close.

Sometimes love
is simply
the one who turns the light on
when she can't find the switch.

The Ones Who Hold Us

No one mother is
on an island.
There are hands
that steady the edges—
a partner who learns the dance
of nappies and midnight shushing,
who brings water
before she even asks,
who sees the tremble
and stays.

There are friends
who drop meals on the doorstep,
who take the toddler's hand
so she can take a breath,
who listen
without fixing.

There are neighbours
who notice the bins,
family who rock the baby
long enough
for a shower or a cry—
whatever comes first.

This is the village:
the quiet love
that lifts her
so she can lift her child.
Mothering is a miracle—
and miracles
are never done
alone.

The Modern Village

They say it takes a village.
But most of us
have apartments,
locked doors,
family far away.

So we build one.
Text by text.
Pram walks with someone
we barely know yet.

A neighbour who waves,
then one day
brings bread.

Not grandmothers and aunties—
but group chats,
clinic rooms,
someone who says
me too.

It's slower now.
Not given—
made.
No drums,
no gathering fire.
Just small lights
across a map
of mothers
keeping each other
afloat.

Part XI

Love That Outlasts

Illness rearranges the story.
Love remains the through line.

The Diagnosis

There are those moments where mothers
receive news
that splits a life in two:
before,
after.
The first thought is
not of themselves,
but of their children—
how to keep showing up,
no matter the cost.

Parenting Through Frailty

Illness rearranges everything.
Appointments and treatments
woven between school runs and
bedtime stories.
A mother's body weary,
but her spirit relentless—
still tying shoelaces,
still packing lunches,
still kissing foreheads goodnight.

The children do not always notice.
To them, love looks the same—
a story read aloud,
a hand brushed across their hair,
a smile across the dinner table.

But I notice.
I notice the courage it takes
to keep offering ease
when the body begs for rest.

The Fear of Absence

It is not death itself I fear most,
but absence.
The thought of them growing tall
without my voice guiding them,
without my hand steadying theirs.

I wonder who will teach them
the small things:
how much vegemite to balance the cheese,
how to hold their breath before diving,
how to forgive themselves
when they fall short.

I imagine their milestones without me—
first heartbreak,
graduations,
weddings,
children of their own.
I want to stretch my love so wide
that it wraps around their whole lives,
even when I cannot.

The Legacy We Leave

Legacy is not possessions.
It is the lullabies sung in the night,
the rhythm of footsteps beside them
on the walk to school,
jokes laughed at a hundred times over.

It is the love stitched into ordinary days
that becomes memory without trying.
The smell of my baking,
the echo of my prayers,
the way I said their name
like a blessing.

These are the fingerprints
I hope will remain on them.
Small inheritances of love,
lasting longer than breath.

The Quiet Courage

Parenting with illness
is an act of defiance.
To keep showing up,
even when the body falters.
To keep smiling,
even when the heart shakes.

Some days it feels like despair.
Other days,
like victory.

But always—
it is love,
translating itself into whatever form is left.
Even in frailty,
a mother's love is strong enough
to steady a child's world.

Borrowed Time

I count differently now.
Not in years,
but in seasons.
How many summers to watch them run barefoot?
How many winters to wrap them in scarves
and "bop" their pink noses?

The numbers frighten me.
So I return to the present—
to the curl of a child's hand around mine,
to the laughter that spills across the table,
to the story told with shining eyes,
bright and fleeting,
a song I want to carry into eternity.

Time may be shortened,
but love stretches.
Love does not obey calendars.
It imprints itself into them
in ways they will not even recognise
until years later.

The Secret Grief

There is a quiet grief
for what I may miss—
birthday candles,
teenage midnights,
faces at twenty or thirty that I may not see.
It rises when I tuck them in,
when I watch their sleeping mouths,
when I measure their growing feet.
Grief does not cancel joy.
It brightens it—
because I know it is finite.
Every ordinary day,
a miracle.
Every moment to be their mother,
a gift.

As Long as I am Here

I count the moments
not in years
but in mornings—
the way light lands
on your hair,
the sound of your laugh
bouncing off the walls.

I do not know
how long I have,
only that I have *now*—
your hand in mine,
your breath against my cheek,
your future blooming
in my sightline.

Some say this is unfair.
They are right.
And still—
love finds a way
to keep showing up.
Every kiss
a legacy,
every story
a thread I leave
for you to follow.

When the day comes
that you walk further
than my body can go,
I hope you feel it—
how I spent my life
loving you
longer than I lived.

Leaving Traces

I think often about what will remain.
Not my notes,
not my work,
not even my body.
But the traces woven into them.
Off-key songs in a warm kitchen.
Perfume that lingers on a jumper.
Handwriting that wraps a name in love.
One day these will be memories.
Today they are presence.
Perhaps that is enough—
to leave so much love
that even in my absence
they do not feel alone.

The Courage to Tell the Truth

How much should they know?
Protect or prepare—
the ache is that I want both.
So I choose honesty,
wrapped in gentleness.
"I may not always be here,
but my love will not end.
It will live in you,
always."
And I pray that those words
will steady them in ways
my arms someday cannot.

What You Leave With Me, My Mum

I will not remember
every detail—
not the medicines,
not the waiting rooms,
not the way the world
turned unfamiliar
for a while.

But I will remember
how you held me—
the warmth,
the certainty,
the way your love
made space
for my whole self
to grow.

I will remember
your laugh,
your stories,
the sunshine you tucked
into my pockets
for later.

People will say
you are gone.

But I will feel you
in the way I care
for others,
in the courage
I borrow
when I don't think I have any,
in the softness
I offer the world.

You taught me this:
love outlives
the body.

And everywhere I go,
I carry you
forward.

Letter for the Days I May Miss

My loves,
if there comes a day when I am not beside you,
know this: I am still with you.
Not in the way you want,
not in the way I want,
but in ways that will not leave you.

I am in the way you laugh
at something ridiculous and small.
I am in the way you stir soup
and taste it slowly,
deciding when it's "just right."
I am in the songs you hum without realising,
the lullabies I once sang into your hair.

When you feel the sun on your face,
I am there.
When you cry into your pillow,
I am there.
When you doubt yourself,
I am the voice that whispers—
you are more than enough.
You always were.

I grieve the milestones I may miss—
the school concerts,
the heartbreaks,
the weddings,
the children you may one day hold.

But I will not miss you,
because loving you is not something
that ends.

If you carry anything of me,
let it be this:
that I loved you with a love unmeasured,
a love that refused the boundaries of time.
That even if my arms are not there,
my love still holds you.
Always.

Part XII

Other Ways Home

There are many ways to become a mother.
All of them begin with love.

Mothering Beyond Birth

Not every mother
births a baby.

Some come by adoption,
some through another's carrying—
longed for
across distance and time.

Love does not wait
for biology.
It arrives complete,
sure of its belonging,
claiming a child
the moment
their story
threads together.

Surrogacy

Some mothers first
hold their babies
with arms and hearts
still healing.
No scar—
perhaps no milk—
but love,
fierce and undeniable.
Motherhood is not only
what the body does;
it is what the heart
insists on,
what the soul claims
as its own.

Adoption

I have seen a mother meet her baby
through another woman's generosity—
a body stretched,
a season offered,
a gift almost beyond comprehension.
Lives reshaped.

She did not give birth,
but she was born that day—
through another woman's grace,
through the ache of letting go.
And when the child was placed
into her arms,
something ancient recognised itself.

No hesitation,
no question of belonging.

Love recognises love.

Carried by Two Hearts

Sometimes,
the road to a child
takes more than one mother,
more than one body
doing the holy work
of making a life.

One offers the space
to grow,
the other the space
to belong.

Love is not divided—
it multiplies.
A child held
by many hearts
is never unsure
of their worth.

Induced Lactation

I have watched women coax milk
from breasts that
never carried a pregnancy.

Each drop hard-won,
each feed a small miracle.
Love refuses "impossible."

It sits at pumps at midnight,
counts millilitres like prayer,
and calls every glistened bead
sacred.

It is proof that nurture is not bound
to the history of a womb,
but to the persistence of love.

Stepping In

She didn't arrive
at the first chapter—
but she holds herself open
for every page
still to come.

Some love grows quietly,
patient and steady,
learning the language
of a child
who wasn't hers
until she decided
she would stay.

There is courage
in showing up
mid-story
and choosing
family.

Guardians of Growth

They open their doors
and their hearts
to a child whose story
is still unfolding,
whose trust
has been tested
too many times before.

They offer safety first,
love slowly,
patience always.

To foster
is to believe
that every child
deserves a soft place
to land
while their future
finds them.

One Set of Hands

There is one chair
that never stays empty—
though its keeper
rarely sits.

Her hands are always moving,
turning chaos into comfort,
tiredness into tenderness.

She carries every name,
every need,
every late-night question
in a single, steady heart.

They call it solo.
But it is not.

I see it clearly:
this is a whole family
held together
by courage.

It is a constellation—
one light
holding many.

Roots and Wings

They thought
their child-raising years
were behind them—
yet here they are,
packing lunches,
reading bedtime stories,
showing up
again.

Love returns
to the beginning,
offering roots
and wings
at the same time.

Grandparent,
parent,
anchor—
all in one.

Belonging, Doubled

Some families
rewrite the template—
more hearts,
more home,
more ways
to belong.

Two mums
holding one future,
two voices
cheering first steps,
two souls
teaching that love
is the only thing
that defines a family.

Here,
every child
is exactly
where they were meant
to land.

The Mentor Mothers

Some women
mother the world.
They are the ones
who answer the late-night messages,
who show up at the door
with food and knowing eyes,
who teach the latch,
the breath,
the art of staying.

Their arms have held
so many stories—
their own,
and those handed to them
in whispered fear
or quiet hope.

They do not claim
the children they guide,
but they stand steady
as those families
find their way.

Not by blood,
but by devotion—
they are mothers, too.

Mothers of courage,
of community,
of the next generation
of love.

The Many Doors

There is no single doorway into motherhood.
Some walk through birth,
others through loss,
others through the gift of another.
On the far side of every door
the work is the same:
to love,
to protect,
to be undone and remade.

Unexpected Journeys

Family is not always built
the way we imagined.
Sometimes it arrives sideways,
through loss or gift or chance.
But however it comes,
a child is always a beginning,
never a lesser love.

Kinship

I have learned that biology is
not the whole story.
Milk and genes shape bodies,
but love and presence
shape belonging.
A mother is not defined by blood,
but by staying—
again and again
until staying writes home
into a child's bones.

Part XIII

The Long Letting Go

Motherhood is a lifelong practice of release. Each goodbye makes room for who they're becoming.

Older Now

There comes a day
when the baby-soft fades,
and the hand you once held tight
slips away too soon.
Motherhood shifts—
less rocking chairs,
more listening,
less carrying bodies,
more carrying hearts.

New Distance

They build worlds without us.
Friends,
secrets,
laughter
we are not part of.
It is ache and wonder—
both.
To watch them unfold,
to know we are
no longer the centre,
and still,
somehow,
the anchor.

The Long Gaze

With older children
the days are less frantic,
the worries deeper.
Who will they become?
Will kindness take root?
Will they remember
the small, steady love
that held them all along?

Still My Child

Even grown,
they come home tired,
or sad,
or lost.
You still know
how to hold them—
not as tightly as before,
just enough to
remind them:
you are mine,
and I am yours,
still.

The Long Letting Go

No one told me motherhood was mostly
letting go.
From the first cut of the cord—
a slow unravelling.
First from my body,
then from my arms,
then from the centre of their world.
Each stage a small death,
and a resurrection too:
I lose one version of my child
to meet another.
It hurts.
It heals.
This is the rhythm of love.

The Weight of Love

No one told me love
could ache like this.
Every fever a
storm
in my own veins,
every fall knocking breath
from my chest.

I thought love was
warmth and joy—
and it is—
but also a
raw,
relentless
tether.

Nights staring
at the ceiling,
prayers whispered
for strength,
for a kind world,
for me to be enough.

First Goodbye

The last breastfeed came quietly—
no ceremony,
no announcement.
One day you didn't ask,
and I didn't offer.
I sat with the ache of it,
mourning and grateful
at once.

School Gate

I kissed you at the gate
and watched you disappear
into a sea of backpacks.
My arms felt empty;
my heart brimmed with pride.
Motherhood is
learning to love
from a distance—
to let go
without losing.

The Last Time

We never notice
the last time—
the last night
they fall asleep
on our chest,
the last morning
their hand reaches up
before their eyes open,
the last time
they need us
to pour the cereal
or tie the shoe
or kiss the bump
better.
The endings
arrive quietly—
a soft fading
instead of a farewell.

Only later
do we turn around
and realise
a whole era
has slipped into memory
while we were busy
living it.

And grief
meets gratitude
in the same breath—
because we were there
for all those ordinary
miracles.

Braver Than Me

You take a step
further than yesterday,
eyes wide,
heart sure—
as if the whole world
is one big invitation.

I smile,
I cheer,
I say go, go, go—
even as a quiet part of me
whispers: stay.

You are braver
than I ever was
at your age.
Braver than I feel
even now.

And I learn
to follow your lead—
to unclench my heart,
to widen the path,
to believe
you were made
for more than my arms.

This is the strange grace
of growing a child:
you teach me courage
by leaving,
a little
at a time.

The Long Arc

Letting go is never once.
It is a thousand
small releases—
the hand you
no longer need,
the bed you
climb from alone,
the secrets you keep.
Each goodbye hurts,
and makes room
for who
you are
becoming.

Letter to My Future Self

One day
they will no longer need me
in the ways they do now.
This is not failure—
it is fruit.
I will bless the distance,
tend the tether,
and keep a lamp in the window.
The holiest ache of all:
to love them toward the horizon,
and stay
their shore.

Part XIV

Milk, Power & Motherhood

To honour the work of feeding is to honour women's labour.
It is to name what has always held the world together.

More Than Milk

They tell us
to feed our babies—
but not here,
not now,
not like that.

They praise the choice
while stripping away
the supports
that make choice real.

Breastfeeding lives
in the crosshairs
of a world
that wants women's bodies
to work
but never complain,
to nourish
but never need,
to serve
but never take space.

And still—
we rise at midnight,
crack ourselves open
to pour out care,
turning softness
into survival.

This is labour.
This is power.
This is resistance
in plain sight.

Breastfeeding
is more than milk.
It is a mother saying:

My body
is my own—
and life begins
right here.

The Ordinary as Political

Breastfeeding is never just about milk.
It is about power.
It is about who gets to choose,
who gets to be supported,
and who is silenced.

Hospitals call it
support.
Governments call it
strategy.
Companies call it
opportunity.
Only mothers know
the weight of those words.

To speak of breastfeeding in this way
is to name the ordinary
as political.
The private
as public.
The body
as powerful.

The Body Reclaimed

Our breasts have been named
too many times
by others.

Shame.
Spectacle.
Sales pitch.

But to feed at the breast
is to reclaim—
to say:
my body,
my child,
my choice.

Unpaid Labour

They call it instinct—
as if instinct
doesn't cost.
As if the nights
aren't long,
as if the hours
don't stack up,
unrecorded,
unpaid.

Milk is economy.
And we are the workers
whose labour
keeps the world alive
before anyone else wakes.

Still—
no medals,
no wages,
no rest days.

Just the quiet truth:
the smallest mouths
depend
on the biggest effort
no one sees.

Manufactured Doubt

Glossy ads
whisper softly—
you're tired,
you're unsure,
we can fix that.

A bottle,
a promise,
a quiet suggestion
that your body
might not
be enough.

They sell confidence
in tins,
while loosening
your grip
on your own.

And somewhere
between the slogans
and the fear,
a mother forgets
she was born
with wisdom
no company
can trademark.

"I Don't Work"

Breastfeeding is work.
Mothering is work.
Night work.
Day work.
Invisible work.

No wage.
No clock-off.
No applause.

It is the labour
that keeps the world alive.
And it deserves
to be named.

Nights Like These

There were nights
when I thought:
I cannot do this again.

But your small hand
rested on my chest,
and I rose.

Because love
does not wait
for convenience.

Here, In the Light

They ask us
to stay home,
to cover up,
to keep it quiet—
as if nourishment
belongs in the shadows.

But we know
that thriving babies
require brave mothers
in bright spaces.

So we feed
in cafés,
in parks,
in third-row seats
at school concerts—
not for spectacle,
but for survival.
Even when our hands shake.

This is not shame.
This is presence.
This is life
made visible
in the light.

Voice and Silence

So many stories
go unheard.

"I wanted to breastfeed,
but I couldn't."

"I wanted to stop,
but no one believed my pain."

We hold these voices
in waiting rooms,
in parks,
in clinics,
in poems.

Listening
is a radical act.

Believing
is a radical act.

Residue

I have sat with mothers
who whispered their grief—
milk they never made,
milk that ran dry too soon.

And I have sat with others
who longed to stop,
but no one saw
their exhaustion.

I carry their words
in my practice,
in my writing,
in my body.

Systems and Structures

Whose leave is paid?
Whose workplace says no?
Whose feeding traditions
were broken
by colonisation?

This is not just personal.
It is policy.
It is justice.
It is survival.

The Riches We Carry

There is wealth
in our breasts—
quiet,
ordinary,
astonishing.

A medicine
made fresh
every hour.
A resource
renewable
with rest
and reassurance.

It could save millions—
in dollars,
yes,
but also
in hospital beds spared,
immune systems steadied,
grief averted,
tiny chests rising
easier.

But this wealth
is overlooked
because it can't be bottled,
branded,
monetised.

It can only be nurtured—
held through the long nights,
protected by community,
respected by systems
that too often rush
or forget.

Still,
it remains—
abundant,
human,
ancient.

A quiet fortune
that mothers carry
in their bodies,
and babies
drink
into their bones.

Enough

Stop telling us
we can do it all.
We already have.

The proof is everywhere—
in the dishes
cooling in the sink,
the inbox
that hums past midnight,
the child's breath
against our arm
while we plan
tomorrow.

What we want
is not another reminder
of strength,
but permission
to rest.

Not resilience,
but reciprocity.
Not praise for coping,
but the safety
to stop.

We don't need
to do it all.
We need a world
that stops
asking us to.

Not Here to Prove

We have held
too much—
babies, deadlines,
other people's comfort.
We have smiled
through exhaustion
and called it grace.

Now,
we are unlearning.
We are trading
efficiency
for presence,
applause
for ease.

We are allowed
to be tired,
to ask for help,
to rest
without guilt.

This is not surrender.
It is reclamation.
We are not here
to do it all.
We are here
to live it—
fully,
softly,
together.

Whose Choice?

They say
breastfeeding is a choice—
but whose choice
when racism scars care,
when formula marketing
shouts louder
than community,
when support is a privilege—
not a right?

Policy shapes
every latch.
Equity
lets milk flow.

We are not asking
for permission—
we are demanding
a world where breastfeeding
is possible
for every family,
not just the fortunate.

Justice,
like milk,
is meant
to be shared.

Toward Liberation

Imagine a world
where mothers are free.

Free to choose.
Free to be supported.
Free from shame.

Where compassion meets trauma.
Where structures uphold.
Where communities surround.

A future
where breastfeeding
is not burden,
but belonging.

We Are Not Done

We have fed children
in the margins—
behind covers,
behind closed doors,
behind systems
built to silence us.

We have stitched
the safety net ourselves—
with peer support,
with whispered wisdom,
with stubborn survival.

We have carried
a whole economy
on our backs
and called it
love.

But love alone
is not enough
to make justice flow.

We refuse a world
where feeding our children
requires privilege,
permission,
or apology.

We rise
with milk
and knowledge
and an army
of sleepless mothers
who know
that the future
begins here—
at the breast,
in the dark,
with a courage
no one sees
until it changes
everything.

Each drop of milk
is both nourishment
and protest—
a reminder
that what keeps the world alive
has always been women's work.

This is the work.
This is the movement.
This is the revolution
in our bones.

We are not done.
We are just
beginning.

Epilogue

This book is not just mine.
It belongs to every mother I have known,
sat with, wept with, laughed with,
and every mother I will never meet.

It belongs to those who cradle babies,
and those who grieve empty arms.
To those who advocate loudly,
and those who carry the quiet heroism
of ordinary days.

It belongs to the clinicians
who sit gently
with the hardest stories.

It belongs to the mothers
who love,
who endure,
who ache,
who become.

We are never alone in this story.

We never were.

Acknowledgements

My deep thanks to the families who have trusted me with their stories — your courage and tenderness are the heart of this book.

To my own family for the love that steadies me: Imad, Zayn, and Meryem.

To the line of mothers who made me: my Mum, whose determination taught me strength and made so much possible; and my Nanna, whose quiet goodness still lights my way.

To my colleagues and mentors in Breastfeeding and Lactation Medicine, and to the Academy of Breastfeeding Medicine (ABM) and the Breastfeeding Medicine Network of Australia & New Zealand (BMNANZ) for the community and vision you bring.

To the teachers who reminded me that evidence and tenderness belong together; and to all of my loved ones who keep the kettle on.

This book was written in the margins of ordinary days — thank you to everyone who made those margins a little wider.

About the Author

Dr Melody Jackson is an Australian GP and International Board Certified Lactation Consultant (IBCLC) in Sydney, and the founder of Breastfeeding & Beyond, a Breastfeeding and Lactation Medicine (BFLM) practice dedicated to consent-based, trauma-informed care for lactating parents and infants. She serves on the boards of the Academy of Breastfeeding Medicine and the Breastfeeding Medicine Network of Australia & New Zealand, working to strengthen education, research and advocacy for the emerging specialty of Breastfeeding & Lactation Medicine.

In clinic rooms and living rooms, Melody's work traces the places where evidence and tenderness belong together — helping families navigate beginnings and losses, milk and medicine, advocacy and the many transitions that happen as their babies grow. She teaches widely, mentors clinicians, and writes to honour the ordinary heroism of parents who keep showing up.

She is a mother of two, which means her writing mostly started in the "Notes" section of her phone, and is often shaped by school gates, night wakings that have lasted long beyond the newborn period, and the lamp left on in the hallway.

This is her first collection.

Further Support & Resources

If you are struggling or this book brings difficult emotions: Please reach out. You do not have to carry it alone.

Australia:
• PANDA (Perinatal Anxiety & Depression Australia) — 1300 726 306 | panda.org.au
• Lifeline — 13 11 14 | lifeline.org.au
• Beyond Blue — 1300 22 4636 | beyondblue.org.au

International:
• Postpartum Support International (PSI) — +1 800 944 4773 | postpartum.net

If you are in crisis or feel unsafe, please contact your local emergency service.

Your wellbeing matters. You are not alone in your story.

www.ingramcontent.com/pod-product-compliance
Lightning Source LLC
LaVergne TN
LVHW101615210926
848480LV00010B/1027
9781764318310